Aging Backward

Your Holistic Handbook for

Timeless Beauty

Introduction

In a world that often fixates on youth and the relentless pursuit of unblemished skin and boundless vitality, the concept of aging can be misconstrued. It is paramount to acknowledge that aging is an inherently natural and exquisite facet of life—a voyage characterized by life experiences, personal growth, and ever-evolving wisdom. Instead of opposing the flow of time, we have the power to embrace it with elegance and celebrate the profound wisdom it imparts.

" Aging Backward: Your Holistic Handbook for Timeless Beauty" transcends the conventional narratives of averting wrinkles or striving for perpetual youth. It embarks on a profound exploration into the art of graceful aging—a journey where we nourish not only our physical selves but also our minds and spirits, all while safeguarding the vitality and vigor of our skin. This book invites us to embrace the path of aging as a metamorphic odyssey, one that allows us to uncover our most authentic selves.

As we tread the path toward timeless beauty and a perpetual youthful glow, we traverse a landscape rich in wisdom, scientific insights, and holistic philosophies. While aging is an inevitable facet of life, there exists a multitude of avenues through which we can embrace it gracefully, while simultaneously preserving the health and vibrancy of our skin, body, and mind. Within the pages of this comprehensive guide, we embark on a transformative journey through 100 invaluable anti-aging tips that span the realms of skincare, nutrition, exercise, and lifestyle choices. Whether you find yourself in your twenties, keen on averting premature aging, or in the golden years, striving to retain your vitality, these tips shall illuminate the path towards a more youthful and resplendent version of yourself.

1. Stay Hydrated for Youthful Skin

Water is the essence of life, and its importance extends to maintaining youthful skin. When your body is adequately hydrated, your skin appears plump, smooth, and radiant. Water helps flush out toxins and waste products, promoting clear skin and reducing the risk of acne and other skin issues. Dehydration can lead to dryness, flakiness, and even exacerbate the appearance of wrinkles and fine lines.

To maintain proper hydration, aim to drink at least eight 8-ounce glasses of water a day. Adjust your intake based on your activity level, climate, and individual needs. Besides water, incorporate hydrating foods like watermelon, cucumber, and oranges into your diet. These fruits are not only delicious but also help replenish your body's water content.

Additionally, consider using hydrating skincare products, including moisturizers and serums with ingredients like hyaluronic acid, glycerin, and ceramides. These compounds lock in moisture and maintain skin's natural barrier function.

2. The Magic of Fruits and Vegetables

Fruits and vegetables are nutritional powerhouses that provide essential vitamins, minerals, antioxidants, and fiber necessary for healthy skin and overall well-being. These foods are packed with vitamins like A, C, and E, which help combat free radicals that can accelerate aging. They also contain water, which contributes to hydration and skin plumpness.

Leafy greens such as spinach and kale are rich in vitamin K, which plays a role in reducing dark circles under the eyes. Carrots and sweet potatoes provide beta-carotene, a precursor to vitamin A, promoting healthy skin cell turnover. Citrus fruits like oranges and grapefruits offer vitamin C, vital for collagen production and skin repair.

Furthermore, fruits and vegetables are high in dietary fiber, which aids digestion and promotes a healthy gut microbiome. A balanced gut contributes to clear skin and may reduce the risk of skin conditions like acne.

To harness the magic of fruits and vegetables, aim to fill half your plate with these colorful, nutrient-dense foods at every meal. Experiment with different varieties to ensure you receive a wide spectrum of vitamins and minerals.

3. Embrace Healthy Fats for a Glowing Complexion

Healthy fats are essential for skin health and overall anti-aging. Omega-3 fatty acids, found in fatty fish like salmon, walnuts, and flaxseeds, play a crucial role in maintaining skin's lipid barrier. This barrier keeps moisture in and harmful irritants out, preventing dryness, redness, and inflammation.

Monounsaturated fats, present in avocados, olive oil, and nuts, provide skin with essential fatty acids, promoting suppleness and radiance. They also contain vitamin E, an antioxidant that protects skin from UV damage and supports collagen production.

Including these healthy fats in your diet can lead to soft, glowing skin. Aim to incorporate them into your meals regularly, whether through a drizzle of olive oil on your salad, a handful of almonds for a snack, or a serving of salmon for dinner.

In addition to dietary changes, consider using skincare products with healthy fat components. Look for moisturizers with ingredients like shea butter, avocado oil, and jojoba oil to lock in hydration and maintain skin's natural lipid barrier.

4. Omega-3 Fatty Acids: Your Skin's Best Friend

Omega-3 fatty acids are a specific type of healthy fat that deserves special attention for their skin benefits. These fats are crucial for maintaining the integrity of the skin's cell membranes, helping to keep the skin hydrated and supple.

One of the primary omega-3 fatty acids found in fish oil, eicosapentaenoic acid (EPA), has anti-inflammatory properties. It can help calm skin conditions like acne and reduce redness and irritation.

Another omega-3, docosahexaenoic acid (DHA), supports the skin's barrier function. A strong skin barrier helps lock in moisture, keeping the skin plump and youthful.

Omega-3s also have the potential to protect against sun damage. While they're not a replacement for sunscreen, they may reduce the skin's sensitivity to UV rays and help prevent premature aging caused by sun exposure.

To reap the skin benefits of omega-3s, incorporate fatty fish like salmon, mackerel, and sardines into your diet. If you're not a fan of fish, consider omega-3 supplements like fish oil capsules. Consult with a healthcare provider to determine the right dosage for you.

5. Sugar Reduction: A Sweet Deal for Your Skin

Excess sugar consumption can have detrimental effects on your skin. When you consume sugar, your body undergoes a process called glycation. During glycation, sugar molecules bind to proteins in your body, including collagen and elastin, which are responsible for maintaining skin's elasticity and firmness.

This binding process forms harmful molecules called advanced glycation end products (AGEs). AGEs can lead to the breakdown of collagen and elastin, causing skin to become saggy and wrinkled. In addition, AGEs can promote inflammation, which may exacerbate skin conditions like acne and rosacea.

To reduce the impact of sugar on your skin, limit your intake of high-sugar foods and beverages, especially those with added sugars. Opt for natural sweeteners like honey or maple syrup in moderation, and be mindful of hidden sugars in processed foods.

A diet rich in fruits and vegetables can also help counteract the effects of sugar on the skin, as it provides antioxidants that combat oxidative stress caused by AGEs.

Making these dietary adjustments can result in clearer, more youthful skin by preserving collagen and elastin and reducing inflammation.

6. Processed Foods and Trans Fats: Aging Culprits

Processed foods, particularly those containing trans fats, are among the chief culprits when it comes to premature aging. Trans fats are artificially created fats used to extend the shelf life of many processed foods, including baked goods, snack foods, and fried foods.

Consuming trans fats can increase inflammation in the body, leading to various health issues, including skin problems. They can also lead to oxidative stress, which can accelerate skin aging by damaging collagen and elastin fibers.

Additionally, processed foods often lack the nutrients necessary for skin health, such as vitamins, minerals, and antioxidants. Relying on these foods can deprive your skin of the essential building blocks it needs to stay youthful and vibrant.

To protect your skin from the harmful effects of processed foods and trans fats, focus on a whole-foods-based diet. Emphasize fresh fruits, vegetables, lean proteins, and whole grains while minimizing your intake of processed and fried foods. Reading food labels can help you identify and avoid products containing trans fats.

By making these dietary changes, you can reduce inflammation, support skin health, and slow down the aging process.

7. Lean Proteins: Building Blocks of Youth

Lean proteins are the building blocks of your body, and they play a vital role in maintaining youthful skin. Proteins are made up of amino acids, which are essential for collagen production—a key protein that keeps your skin firm and wrinkle-free.

Collagen production naturally decreases as you age, leading to wrinkles and sagging skin. However, a diet rich in lean proteins can help stimulate collagen production and slow down these effects.

Some excellent sources of lean protein include poultry, fish, tofu, beans, and legumes. These foods provide amino acids like proline, lysine, and glycine, which are particularly important for collagen synthesis.

In addition to incorporating lean proteins into your diet, consider using skincare products containing amino acids or peptides. These ingredients can promote collagen production when applied topically, further supporting skin firmness and elasticity.

By prioritizing lean proteins in your meals and skincare routine, you can provide your skin with the essential components it needs to stay youthful and radiant.

8. Whole Grains: The Fiber of Youthfulness

Whole grains are an essential part of a balanced diet, and their benefits extend to your skin's health and overall vitality. Unlike refined grains, which have had the bran and germ removed, whole grains contain the entire grain kernel, providing fiber, vitamins, and minerals.

Fiber is particularly important for skin health because it aids digestion and promotes a healthy gut microbiome. A balanced gut contributes to clear skin and can reduce the risk of skin conditions like acne.

In addition to fiber, whole grains provide essential nutrients like B vitamins (such as niacin and riboflavin) and minerals (like zinc and magnesium) that support skin health. These nutrients play various roles in skin function, including regulating oil production and protecting against UV damage.

To include more whole grains in your diet, opt for options like brown rice, quinoa, whole wheat pasta, and oats. These grains are not only nutritious but also versatile and delicious. Look for skincare products that contain oat extracts or other whole grain ingredients to enhance your skin's health and appearance.

By choosing whole grains, you can promote youthful skin from the inside out, thanks to their fiber, vitamins, and minerals.

9. Antioxidant Powerhouse Foods

Antioxidants are superheroes for your skin. They are compounds that combat oxidative stress, a process that can accelerate skin aging by causing damage to cells and DNA. Antioxidants help neutralize free radicals, unstable molecules that contribute to premature aging and skin conditions.

Several vitamins and minerals act as antioxidants, including vitamins A, C, and E, selenium, and zinc. Incorporating foods rich in these antioxidants into your diet can significantly benefit your skin.

Vitamin A, for example, supports healthy skin cell production and helps prevent signs of aging. You can find it in foods like sweet potatoes, carrots, and spinach. Vitamin C is essential for collagen production and can be found in citrus fruits, strawberries, and bell peppers. Vitamin E, found in nuts, seeds, and avocado, protects the skin from UV damage and keeps it moisturized.

Selenium, present in Brazil nuts, aids in the skin's natural defense against UV rays. Zinc, found in foods like beans and whole grains, helps maintain healthy skin by regulating oil production and reducing inflammation.

To harness the power of antioxidants, focus on a balanced diet rich in colorful fruits and vegetables, nuts, and seeds. These foods provide a variety of antioxidants that work together to protect and rejuvenate your skin.

In addition to dietary sources, consider using skincare products containing antioxidants like vitamin C or E. These products can enhance your skin's defense against environmental stressors.

By nourishing your body with antioxidant-rich foods and skincare, you can help your skin remain youthful and radiant for years to come.

10. Supplements for Skin Health

While a balanced diet should be your primary source of nutrients, supplements can complement your efforts to achieve optimal skin health. Certain vitamins, minerals, and compounds have shown promise in supporting skin function and appearance.

Here are some supplements to consider:

- **Collagen**: Collagen supplements are available in various forms, including powders, capsules, and drinks. Collagen is a protein that provides structure to your skin, hair, and nails. As you age, collagen production naturally decreases, leading to wrinkles and sagging skin. Collagen supplements may help improve skin elasticity and hydration.

- **Vitamin C**: Vitamin C is essential for collagen synthesis and plays a crucial role in skin repair. It's also a potent antioxidant that can protect your skin from free radical damage. Vitamin C supplements may enhance your skin's overall health and appearance.

- **Coenzyme Q10 (CoQ10)**: CoQ10 is an antioxidant that supports cellular energy production. It can help protect your skin from oxidative stress and reduce the appearance of fine lines and wrinkles. CoQ10 supplements may improve skin texture and vitality.

- **Hyaluronic Acid**: Hyaluronic acid is a molecule that helps maintain skin hydration by retaining water. As you age, your skin's natural hyaluronic acid levels decrease, leading to dryness and the appearance of fine lines. Hyaluronic acid supplements may help keep your skin plump and moisturized.

- **Zinc**: Zinc is a mineral that plays a role in skin health by regulating oil production and reducing inflammation. Zinc supplements may benefit individuals with acne or other skin conditions caused by excess oil or inflammation.

Before adding supplements to your routine, consult with a healthcare provider or dermatologist. They can help you determine which supplements, if any, are appropriate for your skin type and concerns.

Keep in mind that supplements should complement a healthy diet and skincare routine, not replace them. A balanced approach that includes a variety of nutrients from whole foods is key to achieving and maintaining healthy, youthful skin.

11. Establish a Daily Skincare Routine

Consistency is key when it comes to skincare. Establishing a daily skincare routine tailored to your skin type and concerns is essential for maintaining healthy, youthful skin. Your routine should include cleansing, moisturizing, and sun protection.

- **Cleansing**: Choose a gentle cleanser that effectively removes dirt, makeup, and impurities without stripping your skin's natural oils. Cleansing helps prevent clogged pores and acne while maintaining a clean canvas for other skincare products.

- **Moisturizing**: A good moisturizer hydrates your skin, preventing dryness and promoting a smooth complexion. Look for a product suitable for your skin type, whether it's dry, oily, or sensitive.

- **Sun Protection**: Apply sunscreen with at least SPF 30 every morning, even on cloudy days. Sunscreen is your first line of defense against UV rays, the primary cause of premature aging. It helps prevent wrinkles, sunspots, and skin cancer.

12. Use a Gentle Cleanser for Makeup Removal

Removing makeup at the end of the day is crucial for healthy skin. However, harsh makeup removers can irritate the skin. Opt for a gentle makeup remover or micellar water that effectively dissolves makeup without tugging or rubbing.

Avoid scrubbing or using abrasive materials on your skin to remove makeup, as this can cause micro-tears and damage.

13. Sunscreen: Your Shield Against Aging Rays

Sunscreen is one of the most vital components of your anti-aging arsenal. UV rays from the sun break down collagen and elastin fibers, leading to sagging skin, wrinkles, and sunspots. Sunscreen protects your skin from these harmful effects.

- **Broad-Spectrum Sunscreen**: Choose a broad-spectrum sunscreen that protects against both UVA and UVB rays. UVA rays prematurely age the skin, while UVB rays cause sunburn.

- **Application**: Apply sunscreen to all exposed areas of your skin, including your face, neck, décolletage, and hands. Don't forget your ears and lips.

- **Reapplication**: Reapply sunscreen every two hours, especially when outdoors or swimming. Sunscreen can wear off, so consistent reapplication is essential.

14. Broad-Spectrum Sunscreen: Defending Against UV Damage

Broad-spectrum sunscreen is your shield against the damaging effects of UV radiation. UVA rays penetrate the skin's deeper layers, causing premature aging and skin cancer. UVB rays primarily affect the skin's surface and are responsible for sunburn.

Broad-spectrum sunscreen safeguards your skin from both UVA and UVB rays, providing comprehensive protection against photoaging and skin cancer.

When choosing a broad-spectrum sunscreen, consider your skin type and any specific concerns you may have, such as sensitivity or acne-prone skin. Look for a product that suits your needs and has an SPF rating of at least 30 for daily use.

15. Sunscreen Application: A Non-Negotiable Habit

Applying sunscreen daily is a non-negotiable skincare habit for maintaining youthful skin. UV radiation is a potent accelerator of skin aging, causing wrinkles, fine lines, and sunspots.

To effectively protect your skin:

- **Apply Generously**: Use enough sunscreen to cover all exposed areas of your skin thoroughly. A thin application may not provide adequate protection.

- **Cover All Exposed Skin**: Don't forget areas like your neck, ears, and the back of your hands. UV damage can occur even in seemingly small or hidden areas.

- **Apply 15 Minutes Before Sun Exposure**: Give your skin time to absorb the sunscreen before heading outdoors.

- **Reapply Every Two Hours**: Sunscreen can wear off, especially if you're sweating or swimming. Reapplication ensures continuous protection.

16. Antioxidants in Skincare: Age-Defying Allies

Antioxidants are powerful age-defying allies for your skin. They combat free radicals, unstable molecules that can cause skin damage and accelerate aging. Common antioxidants used in skincare include vitamins C and E, green tea extract, and resveratrol.

Incorporating antioxidant-rich skincare products into your routine can help neutralize free radicals, reduce inflammation, and promote a youthful complexion. Look for products with proven antioxidants and include them in both your morning and evening routines.

17. Retinol (Vitamin A): The Wrinkle Warrior

Retinol, a form of vitamin A, is a potent ingredient for reducing wrinkles and fine lines. It promotes collagen production, improves skin texture, and helps fade age spots and sun damage. Retinol can also unclog pores, making it beneficial for acne-prone skin.

When using retinol, start with a lower concentration to allow your skin to acclimate. Apply it at night and use sunscreen during the day, as retinol can increase sun sensitivity. Over time, you can gradually increase the concentration if needed.

18. Moisturization: Your Skin's Best Friend

Moisturizing is a fundamental step in any skincare routine. It helps maintain skin hydration, preventing dryness, flakiness, and irritation. Properly hydrated skin appears plump, smooth, and youthful.

Choose a moisturizer suitable for your skin type, whether it's lightweight for oily skin or richer for dry skin. Apply it consistently after cleansing to lock in moisture and support your skin's natural barrier function.

19. Exfoliation: Renewing Skin's Youthful Glow

Exfoliation is the process of removing dead skin cells from the surface of your skin. It helps improve skin texture, reduce the appearance of fine lines, and promote a youthful glow. There are two main types of exfoliation: physical and chemical.

- **Physical Exfoliation**: Physical exfoliants contain small particles or ingredients like sugar or jojoba beads that physically slough off dead skin cells when massaged onto the skin. Use these products with gentle, circular motions to avoid irritation.

- **Chemical Exfoliation**: Chemical exfoliants contain alpha hydroxy acids (AHAs) or beta hydroxy acids (BHAs) that dissolve dead skin cells. AHAs are water-soluble and work on the skin's surface, while BHAs are oil-soluble and can penetrate pores. Chemical exfoliants can be milder than physical exfoliants and are often recommended for sensitive skin.

Exfoliate no more than 2-3 times a week to avoid overdoing it, which can lead to irritation. Always follow exfoliation with moisturizer and sunscreen, as exfoliated skin is more susceptible to sun damage.

20. The Importance of Restful Sleep

Quality sleep is essential for skin health and overall well-being. During deep sleep, your body repairs and regenerates cells, including skin cells. Lack of sleep can lead to puffy eyes, dark circles, and dull skin.

To promote restful sleep:

- **Establish a Routine**: Go to bed and wake up at the same time each day to regulate your body's internal clock.

- **Create a Relaxing Bedtime Ritual**: Wind down before bed with activities like reading, gentle stretching, or taking a warm bath.

- **Limit Screen Time**: Reduce exposure to screens, as the blue light emitted can disrupt sleep patterns.

- **Create a Comfortable Sleep Environment**: Ensure your bedroom is dark, quiet, and at a comfortable temperature.

Prioritizing sleep is an essential part of your anti-aging strategy, as it allows your skin and body to rejuvenate, resulting in a fresher and more youthful appearance.

These are the next set of tips in our comprehensive guide to anti-aging. Each of these points addresses a specific aspect of skincare and lifestyle that can contribute to maintaining youthful, healthy skin. By following these tips, you can establish a solid foundation for your anti-aging routine and work toward achieving your skin goals.

21. Stress Management: Your Elixir of Youth

Chronic stress can accelerate the aging process and take a toll on your skin's health. Stress triggers the release of cortisol, a hormone that can break down collagen and elastin, leading to wrinkles and sagging skin. Additionally, stress can exacerbate skin conditions like acne and eczema.

Effective stress management techniques, such as meditation, yoga, deep breathing exercises, and mindfulness, can help reduce stress levels and promote overall well-being. Prioritize self-care practices that relax your mind and body to keep your skin youthful.

22. Quit Smoking, Limit Alcohol

Smoking is a major contributor to premature aging. It narrows blood vessels, reducing blood flow to the skin and depriving it of essential nutrients. Smoking also damages collagen and elastin, leading to wrinkles and a dull complexion. Quitting smoking is one of the best anti-aging choices you can make for your skin and overall health.

While moderate alcohol consumption is generally considered safe, excessive drinking can dehydrate your skin and dilate blood vessels, leading to redness and broken capillaries. Limit alcohol intake and stay hydrated to minimize its potential effects on your skin.

23. Stay Active: The Fountain of Youth

Regular physical activity is often called the fountain of youth for good reason. Exercise improves circulation, delivering oxygen and nutrients to skin cells, promoting collagen production, and aiding in the removal of waste products. It also helps reduce stress, which can have positive effects on your skin.

Aim for at least 150 minutes of moderate-intensity aerobic exercise or 75 minutes of vigorous-intensity exercise per week, as recommended by health authorities. Incorporate activities you enjoy, whether it's walking, jogging, swimming, or dancing.

24. Regular Medical Check-Ups: Early Prevention

Regular check-ups with your healthcare provider are crucial for early detection and prevention of health issues that can impact your skin and overall well-being. These appointments can catch potential problems early, allowing for prompt treatment and better outcomes.

Be sure to discuss any skin concerns or changes during your check-ups, as your healthcare provider can provide guidance or refer you to a dermatologist if needed.

25. Maintain a Healthy Weight

Maintaining a healthy weight is essential for overall health, including skin health. Excess weight can lead to a variety of skin problems, including chafing, stretch marks, and skin infections. Moreover, it can increase the risk of conditions like diabetes, which can negatively affect skin health.

Achieving and maintaining a healthy weight through a balanced diet and regular exercise can help you look and feel your best, supporting youthful skin and vitality.

26. Social Connection: The Heart of Longevity

Social connections and strong relationships are associated with longer life and better overall health, which includes healthier, more youthful-looking skin. Meaningful social interactions can reduce stress, boost mood, and improve self-esteem—all factors that contribute to youthful skin.

Make an effort to nurture your social connections, whether through spending time with loved ones, joining clubs or organizations, or participating in social activities that bring you joy.

27. Posture: Stand Tall and Proud

Good posture not only promotes physical well-being but can also enhance your appearance and how you feel about yourself. Slouching or poor posture can lead to muscle imbalances and the appearance of sagging skin.

To maintain good posture, imagine a string pulling you gently upward from the top of your head. Keep your shoulders back and down, and engage your core muscles. Over time, improved posture can contribute to a more confident and youthful presence.

28. Sunglasses: Shields for Timeless Eyes

Sunglasses do more than just make a fashion statement—they protect your eyes from harmful UV rays. Prolonged sun exposure without eye protection can lead to cataracts, macular degeneration, and wrinkles around the eyes.

Look for sunglasses that offer 100% UVA and UVB protection to shield your eyes and the delicate skin around them from UV damage.

29. Eye Care: Vision for Life

Eye health is integral to a youthful appearance. Common eye issues, like dryness, redness, and dark circles, can make you look older than you are.

Maintain eye health by:

- **Getting Regular Eye Exams**: Visit an eye care professional for comprehensive eye exams, especially as you age.

- **Using Eye Drops**: For dry or irritated eyes, use artificial tears or lubricating eye drops.

- **Wearing Blue Light Glasses**: If you spend a lot of time in front of screens, consider blue light glasses to reduce eye strain.

30. Cardiovascular Exercise for a Strong Heart

Cardiovascular exercise, such as brisk walking, running, cycling, and swimming, is essential for heart health. A strong heart pumps blood more efficiently, delivering oxygen and nutrients to your skin and other organs.

Regular cardiovascular exercise helps improve blood circulation, which can give your skin a healthy, rosy glow. It also supports overall health and longevity.

These are the next set of anti-aging tips in our comprehensive guide. Each tip addresses a specific aspect of skincare, lifestyle, or health that can contribute to maintaining youthful, healthy skin. By following these tips, you can continue building a strong foundation for your anti-aging routine and work toward achieving your skincare goals.

31. Healthy Hair Care for a Youthful Look

Healthy hair can enhance your overall appearance and contribute to a youthful look. Proper hair care includes using mild shampoos and conditioners, avoiding excessive heat styling, and protecting your hair from the sun.

Additionally, maintaining a balanced diet rich in vitamins and minerals can promote healthy hair growth and reduce the risk of hair thinning or loss.

32. Dental Care: The Gateway to Youthful Smiles

A bright, healthy smile is a key component of a youthful appearance. Regular dental check-ups, brushing, flossing, and avoiding excessive consumption of staining foods and beverages can help maintain your teeth's health and whiteness.

Consider professional teeth whitening if you're concerned about tooth discoloration, and always wear a mouthguard if you grind your teeth at night to prevent premature wear.

33. Hormone Balance and Skin Health

Hormone imbalances, particularly in women during menopause, can affect skin health. Changes in hormone levels can lead to skin dryness, loss of elasticity, and increased wrinkles.

Consult with a healthcare provider to discuss hormone replacement therapy or other treatments that can help balance hormones and support healthier, more youthful skin.

34. Sleep Position: Wrinkle Prevention

Your sleep position can affect the formation of wrinkles. Sleeping on your side or stomach can lead to the development of sleep lines, which can become permanent over time.

To minimize wrinkles, consider sleeping on your back. You can also use a silk or satin pillowcase, which creates less friction on your skin compared to cotton, reducing the risk of sleep lines.

35. Collagen-Boosting Foods

Collagen is a protein that provides structural support to the skin, keeping it firm and wrinkle-free. Consuming foods rich in collagen-boosting nutrients can help maintain youthful skin.

Some of these nutrients include vitamin C, which supports collagen production, and amino acids like proline, lysine, and glycine, which are essential for collagen synthesis. Foods like citrus fruits, bell peppers, and bone broth contain these nutrients and can support your skin's collagen production.

36. Regular Hair Trims for Healthy Locks

Regular hair trims can help maintain the health and appearance of your hair. Trimming removes split ends and prevents them from traveling up the hair shaft, leading to breakage and frizz.

How often you should trim your hair depends on your hair type and the rate of growth. Generally, a trim every 6-8 weeks is a good guideline to follow.

37. Mindful Makeup Removal

Removing makeup gently and thoroughly is essential for maintaining healthy skin. Failing to remove makeup can lead to clogged pores and breakouts.

Use a makeup remover or micellar water to dissolve makeup, followed by a gentle cleanser to cleanse your skin. Avoid rubbing or tugging at your skin, especially around the delicate eye area.

38. Lip Care: Smooth and Youthful Lips

The skin on your lips is thinner and more delicate than on the rest of your face, making it susceptible to dryness and wrinkles. To keep your lips smooth and youthful:

- **Hydrate**: Drink plenty of water to keep your lips hydrated from the inside.
- **Lip Balm**: Use a lip balm with SPF to protect your lips from UV damage.
- **Exfoliate**: Gently exfoliate your lips to remove dead skin cells. You can use a homemade sugar scrub or a soft toothbrush.

39. Massage for Relaxation and Skin Health

Regular massages can provide relaxation benefits, reduce stress, and improve circulation. Improved circulation can help deliver essential nutrients and oxygen to the skin, contributing to a healthy, youthful complexion.

Consider incorporating facial massages into your skincare routine to boost circulation and promote a youthful glow.

40. Hydration for Healthy Skin and Hair

Proper hydration is essential for healthy skin and hair. Drinking enough water helps maintain skin's moisture levels, reducing the risk of dryness and flakiness.

Hydrated hair is less prone to breakage and split ends. Ensure you're drinking an adequate amount of water daily, and consider using hydrating skincare and haircare products for added moisture.

41. Scalp Health: The Foundation for Beautiful Hair

A healthy scalp is the foundation for beautiful hair. Scalp issues, such as dandruff or excess oil production, can affect hair health and appearance.

Use a gentle, sulfate-free shampoo and conditioner suitable for your hair type and address any scalp concerns with appropriate treatments or products.

42. Gentle Hair Styling Practices

Overly tight hairstyles or constant use of hair accessories like rubber bands can damage your hair and lead to breakage. Opt for looser hairstyles and avoid tying your hair back too tightly.

Also, minimize the use of heat styling tools, and when you do use them, apply a heat protectant spray to shield your hair from damage.

43. Cut Down on Sugary Drinks

Sugary drinks like soda and some fruit juices can negatively impact your skin's health. High sugar consumption can lead to glycation, a process in which sugar molecules bind to proteins in your skin, contributing to the breakdown of collagen and elastin. This can lead to sagging skin and wrinkles.

Opt for water, herbal tea, or naturally flavored water to stay hydrated without the added sugar.

44. Aromatherapy for Relaxation

Aromatherapy involves using essential oils to promote relaxation and reduce stress. Stress reduction can positively impact skin health, as chronic stress can lead to skin issues and accelerate aging.

Incorporate aromatherapy into your routine through methods like diffusers, scented candles, or adding a few drops of essential oil to your bath.

45. Green Tea: An Antioxidant Powerhouse

Green tea is rich in antioxidants, particularly epigallocatechin gallate (EGCG). These antioxidants can help protect your skin from oxidative stress and UV damage, reducing the risk of premature aging.

Enjoy a cup of green tea daily, and consider using skincare products that contain green tea extract for added antioxidant protection.

46. Patience in Skincare: Results Take Time

When starting a new skincare routine or trying different products, remember that results may not be immediate. It can take weeks or even months to see noticeable improvements in your skin.

Be patient and consistent with your skincare routine, and avoid the temptation to switch products frequently. Give your skin time to adjust and respond to the treatments you're using.

47. Cool Showers for Skin Health

Hot showers can strip your skin of natural oils and lead to dryness. Opt for lukewarm or cool showers, especially when washing your face and body. Cooler water can help maintain your skin's natural moisture barrier.

48. Avoid Touching Your Face

Touching your face frequently can transfer dirt, bacteria, and oils from your hands to your skin, potentially leading to breakouts and irritation. Be mindful of this habit, especially if you have a tendency to rest your chin or cheeks on your hands.

49. Consult a Dermatologist

If you have persistent skin concerns or issues that don't respond to over-the-counter treatments, consider consulting a dermatologist. A dermatologist can provide personalized skincare recommendations, prescribe medications, or perform procedures to address your specific needs.

50. Environmental Protection

Protect your skin from environmental factors that can accelerate aging, such as pollution and harsh weather conditions. Consider using skincare products that contain antioxidants and barrier repair ingredients to shield your skin from these stressors.

We're halfway through our comprehensive guide to anti-aging, with each point addressing a specific aspect of skincare, health, or lifestyle that contributes to maintaining youthful, healthy skin. By following these tips, you can continue to build a strong foundation for your anti-aging routine and work toward achieving your skincare goals.

51. Silicon: Support for Healthy Skin and Hair

Silicon is a mineral that plays a role in maintaining healthy skin, hair, and nails. It supports collagen production, which is essential for skin elasticity and youthfulness.

Foods like bananas, whole grains, and leafy greens are good dietary sources of silicon. Additionally, silicon supplements are available, but consult with a healthcare provider before adding them to your routine.

52. Humidifier for Skin Hydration

Using a humidifier in your home, especially during the dry winter months, can help maintain optimal moisture levels in your skin. Adequate indoor humidity can prevent dryness, flakiness, and irritation.

53. Skin Protection During Air Travel

Air travel can dehydrate your skin due to the low humidity levels in airplane cabins. To protect your skin during flights:

- Drink plenty of water to stay hydrated.

- Apply a moisturizer before and during the flight.

- Consider using a hydrating facial mist to refresh your skin.

54. Facial Exercises for Muscle Tone

Facial exercises involve specific movements to target facial muscles. Regular practice may help tone facial muscles, potentially reducing the appearance of sagging skin and wrinkles. These exercises can be particularly useful for the jawline, cheeks, and forehead.

55. Lemon Water for Detoxification

Some people incorporate lemon water into their morning routine for its potential detoxifying effects. While there's limited scientific evidence to support significant detoxification, staying hydrated with lemon water can be a healthy habit that supports overall well-being.

Lemon water provides vitamin C, an antioxidant that can benefit skin health by promoting collagen production.

56. Stress Reduction Techniques

Chronic stress can accelerate aging and negatively impact skin health. Engaging in stress reduction techniques such as yoga, meditation, or deep breathing exercises can help maintain a youthful complexion.

These practices lower cortisol levels, which can reduce the breakdown of collagen and elastin, essential components for firm, youthful skin.

57. Red Light Therapy for Collagen Production

Red light therapy involves exposure to low-level red or near-infrared light. It's believed to stimulate collagen production and improve skin elasticity, potentially reducing the appearance of fine lines and wrinkles.

You can find red light therapy devices for home use or consult a skincare professional for treatments.

58. Hyaluronic Acid for Skin Hydration

Hyaluronic acid is a naturally occurring substance in the skin that helps retain moisture. Using skincare products containing hyaluronic acid can help keep your skin hydrated, plump, and youthful in appearance.

59. Massage for Lymphatic Drainage

Lymphatic drainage massages can help reduce puffiness in the face and promote lymphatic system health. These massages involve gentle, rhythmic strokes that encourage the natural flow of lymphatic fluid, which carries away waste and toxins.

Regular lymphatic drainage massages can help maintain a more sculpted, youthful facial appearance.

60. Avoid Excessive Alcohol Consumption

Excessive alcohol consumption can lead to dehydration, which can negatively affect your skin's appearance. Limit alcohol intake and stay hydrated with water to maintain skin health.

Alcohol can also dilate blood vessels, leading to redness and facial flushing. Moderation is key for both your skin and overall health.

61. Liposomal Supplements for Skin Health

Liposomal supplements are designed to improve nutrient absorption. Some supplements, such as vitamin C or collagen, are available in liposomal form. These supplements may enhance your skin's access to essential nutrients that support a youthful complexion.

Consult with a healthcare provider before adding any new supplements to your routine.

62. Maintain Healthy Nails

Healthy nails can enhance your overall appearance. To maintain nail health:

- Keep your nails clean and trimmed.
- Avoid excessive use of nail polish and nail polish removers.
- Moisturize your cuticles to prevent dryness and hangnails.

63. Sleep Pillowcases for Hair and Skin

Silk or satin pillowcases can reduce friction on your hair and skin compared to cotton pillowcases. This reduced friction can help prevent hair breakage, split ends, and sleep lines on your face.

Consider investing in silk or satin pillowcases for a gentler sleep experience.

64. Skin-Boosting Supplements

Some supplements are specifically formulated to support skin health. These supplements may contain a combination of vitamins, minerals, and antioxidants that promote youthful skin.

Consult with a healthcare provider or dermatologist before adding skin-boosting supplements to your routine to ensure they're appropriate for your needs.

65. Skin Treatments: Chemical Peels

Chemical peels involve applying a chemical solution to the skin to exfoliate the top layer. This process can improve skin texture, reduce the appearance of fine lines and wrinkles, and address issues like acne scars and sun damage.

Chemical peels should be performed by a licensed skincare professional or dermatologist to ensure safety and effectiveness.

66. Bone Broth for Collagen Support

Bone broth is rich in collagen, a key component for skin elasticity. Consuming bone broth provides collagen and essential amino acids that support skin health.

Consider adding bone broth to your diet as a nutritious way to support youthful skin from the inside out.

67. Facial Oils for Hydration

Facial oils, such as jojoba oil, argan oil, and rosehip oil, can provide intense hydration and nourishment for the skin. These oils can help maintain skin moisture, reduce dryness, and promote a radiant complexion.

Apply a few drops of facial oil after your moisturizer for an extra layer of hydration.

68. Silk Hair Ties for Gentle Hold

Traditional elastic hair ties can cause breakage and damage to your hair. Silk hair ties provide a gentle hold that minimizes hair breakage and creasing.

Consider switching to silk hair ties to protect your hair while keeping it secure.

69. Lavender Oil for Relaxation

Lavender oil is known for its calming and relaxation-inducing properties. Incorporate lavender oil into your bedtime routine to promote restful sleep, reduce stress, and support overall well-being, which can positively impact your skin.

You can use lavender oil in a diffuser, add a few drops to your bath, or apply it topically (diluted with a carrier oil) to your pulse points.

70. Skin-Friendly Sleep Position

The way you sleep can affect the formation of wrinkles. Sleeping on your stomach or side can cause sleep lines to develop over time.

To minimize sleep lines, consider sleeping on your back. This position reduces the pressure on your face and can help prevent wrinkle formation.

These are the next set of anti-aging tips in our comprehensive guide. Each tip addresses a specific aspect of skincare, health, or lifestyle that contributes to maintaining youthful, healthy skin. By following these tips, you can continue to build a strong foundation for your anti-aging routine and work toward achieving your skincare goals.

71. Skin-Enhancing Supplements: Omega-3 Fatty Acids

Omega-3 fatty acids, found in fish oil supplements or foods like salmon and walnuts, can help maintain skin health. These healthy fats support the skin's lipid barrier, keeping it moisturized and reducing the risk of dryness and irritation.

Including omega-3-rich foods in your diet or taking supplements can support a youthful complexion.

72. Embrace Facial Yoga

Facial yoga involves exercises that target facial muscles to improve tone and reduce the appearance of wrinkles. These exercises can be done at home and may help maintain a youthful facial appearance.

Some facial yoga exercises include puffing out your cheeks, lifting your eyebrows, and smiling with your lips closed. Regular practice can potentially yield noticeable results.

73. Alcohol-Free Toner for Balance

A gentle, alcohol-free toner can help balance your skin's pH levels and remove any remaining traces of makeup or cleanser. Toners with soothing ingredients like rosewater or chamomile can be especially beneficial for sensitive skin.

Use a toner after cleansing to prepare your skin for serums and moisturizers.

74. Healthy Fats for Skin Moisture

Incorporate healthy fats into your diet, such as avocados, nuts, and olive oil. These fats provide essential fatty acids that support the skin's natural moisture barrier, helping to prevent dryness and maintain a radiant complexion.

75. Consider Collagen Supplements

Collagen supplements come in various forms, such as powders, capsules, or drinks. They are designed to support skin elasticity, reduce wrinkles, and promote youthful-looking skin.

Before using collagen supplements, consult with a healthcare provider to determine if they are suitable for your skin and overall health.

76. Exfoliating Body Scrub

Just as your face benefits from exfoliation, your body can too. Regular use of an exfoliating body scrub can remove dead skin cells, promote smoother skin, and reduce the appearance of dryness and rough patches.

Use a gentle body scrub 2-3 times a week in the shower for best results.

77. Natural Face Masks

Natural face masks made from ingredients like honey, yogurt, or aloe vera can provide hydration, soothe the skin, and improve its overall condition. Incorporate a weekly face mask into your skincare routine to enhance your skin's radiance.

78. Limit Processed Foods

Processed foods often contain high levels of sugar, salt, and unhealthy fats, which can contribute to inflammation and skin issues. Reducing your intake of processed foods can lead to healthier skin.

Focus on a diet rich in fresh fruits, vegetables, lean proteins, and whole grains for optimal skin health.

79. Gua Sha Facial Massage

Gua Sha is a traditional Chinese facial massage technique that involves using a smooth-edged tool to massage the face. It's believed to promote lymphatic drainage, reduce puffiness, and improve skin circulation.

When performed regularly, Gua Sha can contribute to a more youthful and radiant complexion.

80. Probiotics for Gut Health

Gut health is closely linked to skin health. Probiotics, found in foods like yogurt, kefir, and sauerkraut, can support a healthy gut microbiome. A balanced gut microbiome can help reduce inflammation and promote clear, youthful skin.

Consider incorporating probiotic-rich foods into your diet or taking probiotic supplements as recommended by a healthcare provider.

81. Prevent Tech Neck

Spending long hours looking down at screens can contribute to "tech neck," characterized by horizontal lines and sagging skin on the neck. To prevent tech neck:

- **Maintain Good Posture**: Keep your head up and shoulders back when using devices.

- **Take Breaks**: Take breaks from screen time to stretch your neck and shoulders.

- **Neck Exercises**: Incorporate neck-strengthening exercises into your routine.

82. Coconut Oil for Skin and Hair

Coconut oil is a versatile natural product that can benefit both your skin and hair. It provides deep hydration, reduces the risk of dryness, and can be used as a hair mask to improve hair health and shine.

Apply coconut oil to your skin and hair, leave it on for a short period, and then rinse or wash it off.

83. Chemical-Free Sunscreens

When choosing a sunscreen, opt for products that are free of harmful chemicals like oxybenzone and octinoxate, which can harm coral reefs and potentially irritate your skin.

Look for mineral sunscreens that contain zinc oxide or titanium dioxide as the active ingredients for effective and safe sun protection.

84. Hair Serum for Shine

Hair serums contain ingredients that can add shine and manageability to your hair. Apply a small amount of hair serum to the ends of your hair to reduce frizz and enhance the overall appearance of your hair.

85. Mindful Eating Habits

Practicing mindful eating involves paying attention to what you eat, savoring each bite, and listening to your body's hunger and fullness cues. Mindful eating can help prevent overeating, promote healthy digestion, and support overall well-being, which can positively impact your skin.

Take your time when eating, and focus on the taste, texture, and satisfaction of your meals.

86. Reduce Sugar Intake

High sugar consumption can lead to glycation, a process where sugar molecules bind to proteins in your skin, contributing to the breakdown of collagen and elastin. This can lead to sagging skin and wrinkles.

Reducing your sugar intake by limiting sugary snacks and beverages can support youthful skin.

87. Retinol for Wrinkle Reduction

Retinol is a form of vitamin A that can help reduce the appearance of fine lines and wrinkles. It promotes skin cell turnover and collagen production, leading to smoother, more youthful-looking skin.

Incorporate a retinol-based product into your nighttime skincare routine, and use sunscreen during the day when using retinol.

88. Meditation for Stress Reduction

Meditation is a powerful stress reduction technique that can positively impact your skin. By reducing stress, you lower cortisol levels, which can help prevent the breakdown of collagen and elastin, key components for youthful skin.

Practice meditation regularly to promote relaxation and maintain a youthful complexion.

89. Proper Bra Support

Wearing a well-fitting bra that provides proper support is essential for breast health and maintaining a youthful appearance. A supportive bra can help prevent sagging and discomfort.

Consider getting professionally fitted for a bra to ensure you're wearing the right size.

90. Ice Cubes for Puffy Eyes

If you wake up with puffy eyes, ice cubes can be a quick remedy. Wrap an ice cube in a clean cloth and gently press it to your eyelids for a few minutes. The cold temperature can help reduce puffiness and wake up your eyes.

91. Avoid Overwashing Your Hair

Overwashing your hair can strip it of natural oils, leading to dryness and potential damage. Determine a washing frequency that suits your hair type, whether it's daily, every other day, or less frequently.

Use a gentle, sulfate-free shampoo to minimize damage.

92. Mindful Sun Exposure

While sunlight is essential for vitamin D production and overall well-being, excessive sun exposure can lead to premature aging and skin damage. Practice mindful sun exposure by:

- Wearing sunscreen with at least SPF 30.
- Seeking shade during peak sunlight hours.
- Wearing protective clothing like wide-brimmed hats and sunglasses.

93. Natural Sleep Aids

If you struggle with occasional sleeplessness, consider natural sleep aids like valerian root or chamomile tea. These remedies can help you relax and improve sleep quality, supporting your skin's rejuvenation during rest.

94. Vitamin E for Skin Health

Vitamin E is an antioxidant that can protect your skin from oxidative stress and UV damage. You can find vitamin E in skincare products like serums and creams or incorporate it into your diet through foods like almonds and sunflower seeds.

95. Warm Water for Hair Rinse

When rinsing your hair, use lukewarm water instead of hot water. Hot water can strip your hair of natural oils, leading to dryness and frizz.

Finish your hair rinse with a blast of cold water to seal the hair cuticles and add shine.

96. Skin Stretching: Facial Expressions

Engaging in facial expressions that stretch and contract facial muscles can help improve muscle tone and reduce the appearance of wrinkles. Practice exercises like smiling widely, puckering your lips, and raising your eyebrows.

Consistent practice can contribute to a more youthful facial appearance.

97. Hemp Oil for Skin and Hair

Hemp oil is rich in omega-3 and omega-6 fatty acids, making it a beneficial addition to your skincare and haircare routine. It can moisturize and nourish both your skin and hair, promoting a healthy and youthful look.

Use hemp oil as a moisturizer or hair treatment, either by itself or in products.

98. Include Daily Walk as Part of Your Lifestyle

Daily walking offers a multitude of benefits for both physical and mental well-being. It's a simple yet effective way to boost cardiovascular health, lower the risk of chronic diseases like diabetes and heart disease, and maintain a healthy weight.

Beyond the physical advantages, daily walks provide mental clarity, reduce stress and anxiety, and elevate mood by releasing endorphins. They offer a precious opportunity for reflection, mindfulness, and a connection to nature, fostering a sense of tranquility and overall vitality.

99. Aloe Vera Gel for Skin Irritation

Aloe vera gel is known for its soothing properties. Apply aloe vera gel to irritated or sunburned skin to reduce redness, inflammation, and discomfort. It can promote faster healing and maintain skin health.

100. Antioxidant-Rich Foods

Consume a diet rich in antioxidants to protect your skin from free radical damage. Foods like berries, dark leafy greens, and nuts are high in antioxidants that can support your skin's health and youthfulness.

Include these foods in your meals and snacks to benefit from their skin-protective properties.

Conclusion

As we conclude this journey through 100 anti-aging tips, remember that age is just a number, and your beauty is an enduring reflection of your care and choices. By nurturing your skin, nourishing your body, and embracing a holistic approach to wellness, you can gracefully navigate the path of time. The wisdom shared in this guide is your companion, guiding you towards a future where your radiance continues to shine brightly. May you age not just gracefully, but beautifully, inside, and out.

Disclaimer: The information provided in this e-book is for educational purposes only and should not replace professional medical advice. Please consult with a healthcare provider or qualified specialist before making any significant changes to your diet, exercise routine, or lifestyle, especially if you have underlying medical conditions or specific health concerns.

Final Thoughts:

- **"Do you not know that you are the temple of God and that the Spirit of God dwells in you? If anyone defiles the temple of God, God will destroy him. For the temple of God is holy, which temple you are". (1 Corinthians 3:16-17).**

- 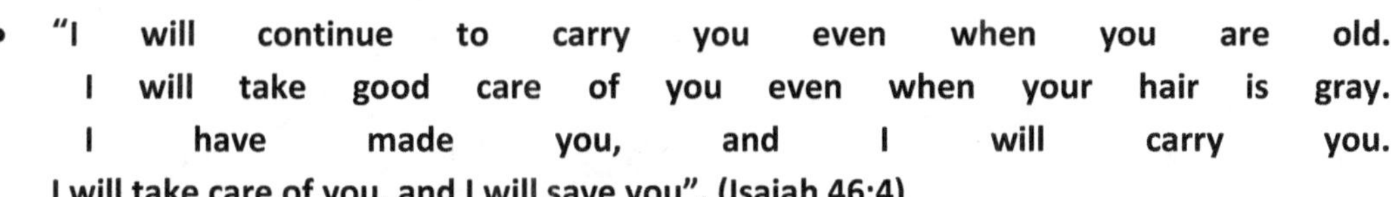 "I will continue to carry you even when you are old. I will take good care of you even when your hair is gray. I have made you, and I will carry you. I will take care of you, and I will save you". (Isaiah 46:4)

www.ingramcontent.com/pod-product-compliance
Lightning Source LLC
Chambersburg PA
CBHW060851260726
48661CB00002B/731